YOUR BRAIN - THE ULTIMATE POWER OF WILL

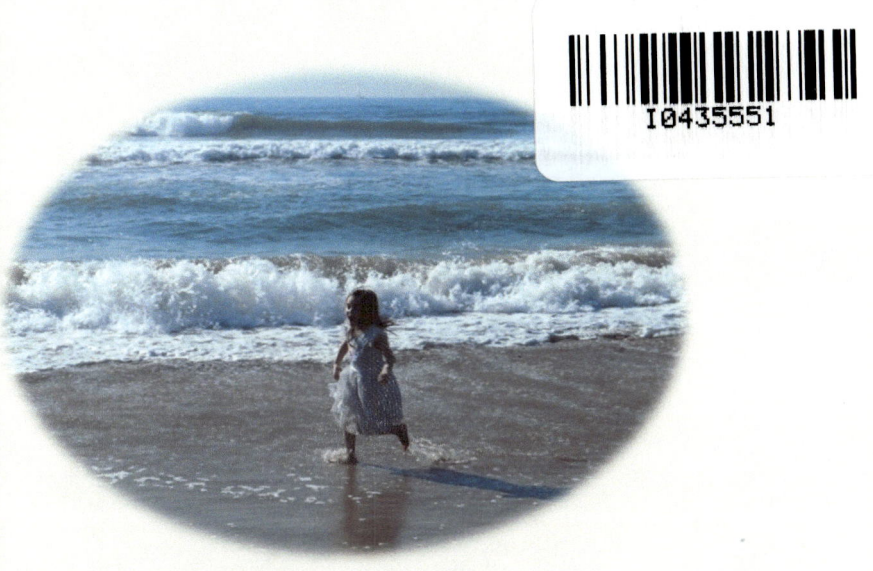

Simple Techniques with Powerful Results

Take Control of Your Body through Your Mind

LaDan Abosein

CONTENTS

INTRODUCTION

Dieting is not about joining a club, or eating or not eating certain foods. It is mostly about understanding your state of mind, finding a comfortable niche for yourself, staying with it for a while, and programming your brain which can respond to certain commands time after time. It is about consistency and perseverance. Not feeling alone when you have all the organs in your body keeping you company and silently urging you to pay more attention to them telling you about their likes and dislikes - when they are overworked and exhausted or underworked and malnourished. Think of a computer programmer who writes codes all day long. Those programming codes unless changed by their creator, always produce the same result which contains series of zeros and ones. Just as a programmer learns to perfect the set of skills with each experience, everything else in life can be pursued with same set of rules and principles.

A key to success in life is to know your objective and staying focused long enough to make it your second nature. Ultimately, you will find your comfort zone which is different for every person and every life style.

I personally stay far away from short term solutions; those promising long and lasting effects. Consider those promises with grain of salt and try to accept them realistically with eyes wide open. Additionally, if you have considered dieting for the purpose of an upcoming event such as a party, a wedding, or summer vacation by the beach realize that you have already limited your brain to an expiration date allowing it to reset after it is over. Consequently, after the already sought after event is over all the bets are off and without a new plan for your brain, it retreats back to its past habits which in this case may be going back to excessive eating since your body is already feeling neglected and deprived of some foods during your dieting phase. Based on our physical body structure, environment, family style and a host of other factors we acquire certain levels of tolerance for hunger and thirst which in some ways define our ability to endure. I call it the power of withstanding hardship, both physical and mental. I for example, have to eat small portions of food every a few hours to maintain certain endurance. According to Merriam-Webster; *endurance is the ability to do something difficult for a long time or the quality of continuing for a long time.* In my opinion the significance of how to maintain our endurance in itself is part of decision making on how to fill our brain and body with either lasting nutrients or short passing impulses. They both sort of do the quick trick but with dramatic long term effects on our body and brain. So the decision is what choice to pursue.

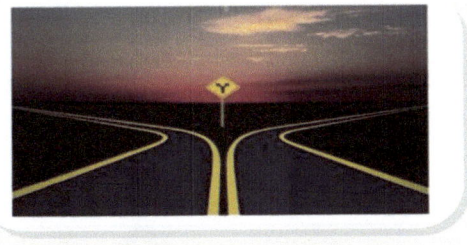

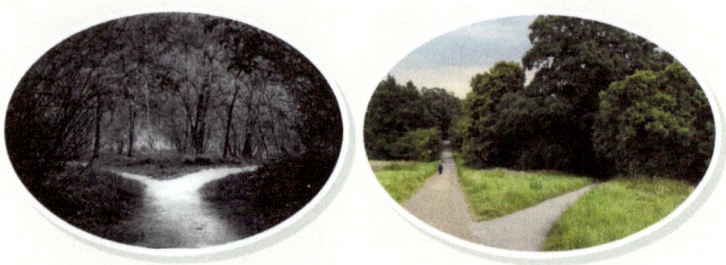

Building a habit that lasts a long time does not happen overnight and certainly is challenging at the least. The first step is to imagine it, define it, develop it in your mind, and nurture it in every fiber of your body and soul so it becomes you; embedded; etched forever and unchangeable unless you decide to change and replace it with something else. In this case, the realization is imprinted in the brain just as series of zeros and ones are coded into the motherboard of a computer delivering the same outputs one hundred percent of the time. Once the program is written and coded into the motherboard the computer doesn't have to think twice before producing the same results to certain commands - it just happens, with stroke of a key. I am talking about the same analogy and mindset when I describe programming your brain to perform certain functions.

A quick checklist:

- ☑ Carry a small pack of food with you at all time.
- ☑ Try to eat as soon as you get the first hunger sign.

☑ Try not to shop on a hungry belly – at least not at the beginning of your programming lessons and not until you feel confident about your ability to manage your impulses.

☑ Relate to fruits and vegetable as your life long best friends – your constant companions that you can literally bite into without getting chewed out.

☑ Find good quality mineral/vitamins or calorie burning supplements from trusted sources as an option. They can be essential part of your sustainability especially if you are maturing with age and your body is experiencing less hormonal activities.

Let's Examine the Recommendations

When pregnant with my daughter I took up the habit of packing small snacks or a sandwich before leaving home. I learned to always keep some type of dried fruit or energy bars in my car. During my pregnancy I sometimes was experienced high fatigue due to a sudden drop in my blood sugar resulting in shakes and shivers. I found the experience very scary as I was walking on a busy street in downtown Chicago or driving the car or riding the train with no immediate access to food or water. From then on I learned to never leave home without having one or two snacks with me. To fight the onset of sudden hunger, some people keep pieces of candy on their person. This is my point exactly by suggesting that advance planning and substituting short lived sugary snacks with something more nutritional and long lasting which contain protein or sweetness of natural fruit, nuts, and vegetable.

Fast forward to today; coming home from work as part of my daily ritual I reach for a large apple which I left that morning on the car seat. Each night as I pack my next day's lunch I put a large apple and napkin into the bag. I leave the apple in the car for my late afternoon snack during the commute home. Chewing my delicious juicy extra-large apple every day makes my driving sweeter and the commuting distance shorter. The real benefit is that I don't have to act impulsive by running to the refrigerator or pantry and reach for something sugary at home. Since we are on the subject of lunch box I also would like to point out the many advantages of packing your own lunch to work. You will find it economically and nutritionally rewarding. For the cost benefit, all you have to do is to add up the daily cost of your trips to fast food restaurants, or vending machines. For the nutritional value, think of the unknown number of calories in addition to the dubious dietary value of the food you're purchasing and consuming every day. I am almost humorously convinced that in order to make certain foods appetizing restaurants sometimes have to add a coat of butter to make their salads shine.

Before leaving the house remember to pack your snack just big enough to fit in your purse, or backpack. For example; slices of cheese, turkey bacon, thin slices of chicken, peanut, or almond butter sandwich, a couple of boiled eggs or a granola bar is among many choices. Keep a bottle of water in your car and drink water instead of any kind of juice or soda. It is easy to justify drinking diet soda instead of water but just because you eliminated the calories it doesn't explain all the other weird ingredients listed on the back of the can or bottle. Act reasonably without going overboard and always remember to explore your own self level of tolerance and limitation.

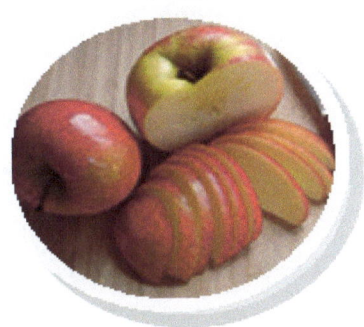

Let's Step onto the Battle-Ground

Weigh the pros and cons of programming your brain and if you decide to proceed with the plan to program your brain get ready for the opposing forces to challenge you on every aspect of your decision; creating obstacles at the emotional and physical level. To combat the opposing forces, learn to:

☑ Eliminate or diminish Temptations and Impulses.

☑ Think of Discipline as Way of Life.

☑ Understand and practice Consistency and what takes to be consistent.

☑ Erase words like *dieting* from your vocabulary.

☑ Learn about Cruise Control mode; relate it to yourself by setting a Rhythm and Speed Pattern which works for you.

☑ Learn how to Reset Your Brain.

☑ Learn how to become one with Your Body.

☑ Learn to explore the Wonders of Your Own Self.

Eliminate or diminish Temptations and Impulses

Life is full of temptations especially when it comes to pleasures such as over spending and eating. It is a life time commitment and continued process of improvement to learn and re-learn the art of sensible spending and eating. The key is to stick with the concept and not to become discouraged with the occurrences of periodic set-backs.

Think of Discipline as Way of Life

Discipline, according to the Merriam Webster is; *A way of behaving that shows a willingness to obey rules or orders. Behavior that is judged by how well it follows set of rules or orders.* So it is all about setting up rules; following those rules to the best of your abilities and remembering that you are your own judge. Also remembering that rules sometimes are meant to be broken and replaced with a new and improved set of rules. The key is to stick with the existing set of rules as long as they are working properly and knowing when to change or tweak them as they become less effective.

Understand the meaning of Consistency and what takes to be consistent

My rule is not to change things as long as they are working properly. This alone makes me to stay with the status quo until I feel it is not working any more. That is my que to put on the thinking cap in pursuant of a different method or tweaking the existing one.

Erase word *dieting* from your vocabulary

Inconsistent pattern of over eating and dieting can result in a series of repeated cycle of weight loss followed by weight gain. However, once you decide not to act impulsive and instead letting you're eating and subsequently all of your habits become influenced by the power of your brain, you'll be surprised by dramatic shift in behavior.

Learn about Cruise Control mode; relate it to yourself by setting a Rhythm and Speed Pattern which works for you

In my experience, repetition works as long as I am satisfied with its outcome. It reminds me of how cruise control in automobiles works; a system that automatically controls the speed of a motor vehicle. The system is a *servomechanism* which maintains a set speed that the driver set and changes with the driver's triggering a change in the already established pattern.

Learn how to Reset Your Brain

Use the wonders of brain to your advantage and unpeel its many complex layers. Recent studies have shown structural changes in human brain after learning a new cognitive skill including vocabulary. Structural neuroplasticity *(increased grey matter volume)* in adults showed an appearance of a qualitative change such as leaning a new task. The neuroscientists' outcome lies beneath the fact that in humans, mental maneuverings can adjust the brain; therefore the neuroplasticity is the mind's ability to change the brain. According to the NIH – *Eunice Kennedy Shriver National Institute of Child health and Human Development:* Based on experiments in animals and humans over the past 20 years, researchers established that the cortex, which is the dominant feature of the human brain, has significant plasticity—the ability to reconfigure its functional organization as the result of experience, such as training. This is supported in animal experiments where a number of physiological changes are observed in response to behavioral training. These include changes in the size and shape of brain regions, speeding up and/or slowing down of neuron signaling, increases in the molecules that help transmit signals through the brain, and the growth of new neurons.

Source: *http://www.nichd.nih.gov/Pages/index.aspx*

Learn how to become one with Your Body

Listen to the wisdom that is already planted in every fiber in your body, just tap-in and listen. Open your heart and mind allowing for the exploration to happen and gradually through cleaning your mind and body you start hearing and feeling the messages. Stop finding excuses for everything and simultaneously stop blaming other factors for your dismays. Listen to the warning signs and analyze them as best as you can. At least be receptive to the messages and avoid dismissing them. Once you open your mind, answers will present themselves and as you open up to receive, they become clearer. Avoid "peer pressure" with all your heart. Sometimes the best approach is the easiest and most obvious one; stop rationalizing and start listening to your inner voices.

Tune into your feelings and listen to your organs as they sometimes communicate to you through aches and pains by showing all kinds of distress.

Learn to explore the Wonders of Your Self

Depending on your age, health, environment, stress level and based on your work and family history among many other elements in your life you may need to adjust you're eating habits. Every five years or so, our hormones along with the shape of our body changes introducing new set of challenges. It is crucial to remain fighter-flexible, keep a sense of humor, be inquisitive, and learn to explore new things. Try to have fun with food and explore all different shapes and forms of the edibles especially the ones whose source is in nature, coming from the ground or trees and bushes. I immediately noticed a change in my body after my 35th birthday. Hormonal changes reduce our bodies' ability to burn calories and we may suddenly show a different reaction to the same food. I haven't always been a healthy eater but I have been a sensible eater and except during my pregnancy I have maintained a certain range in weight and size. Earlier on, if I had to have desert I often substituted a meal for desert by skipping the meal and going right to my favorite chocolate cake or Black Berry pie with a cup of coffee. My rationale by skipping the meal was to save on my calorie intake. However, the day after my 50th birthday I realized that this useless habit had to go. I awakened to the fact that quality food is glorious and necessary for our health and body. I also awoke to the fact that desert is so unnecessary and in my opinion it can be categorized as luxury instead of a necessity. This realization alone was the key to my transformation and for changing my eating habits altogether influencing me to become a walking billboard for sensible eating. I realized something else – we don't need much food to sustain ourselves; just enough to keep us going and the rest is not essential, but habitual. If we learn to master our brain so that when we are suffering from boredom our brain's signaling command be something different than telling us; *hey poor baby you're hungry go feed your hunger or you're really bored therefore you have my permission to gorge* - we may declare a major victory by overcoming our battle of bulges and what is known as impulsive eating. Afterward, we can focus on ourselves and discover what best works for us – I mean the individual us.

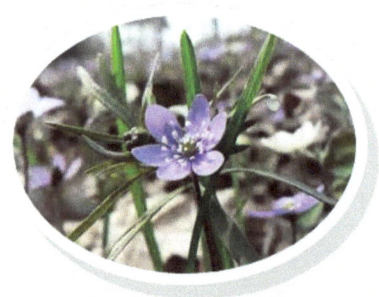

THE BRAIN'S CONTROL CENTER

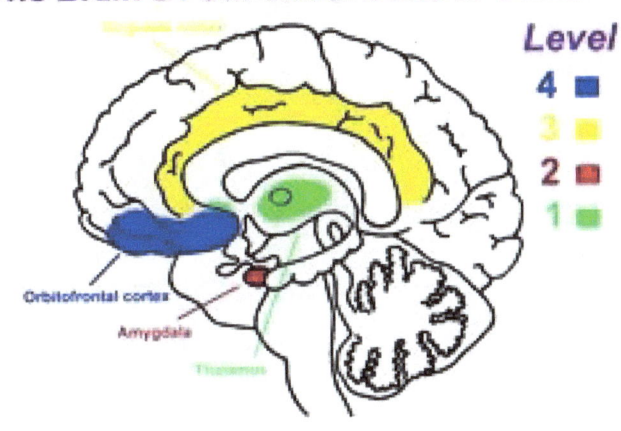

Brain's Control Center

Source: Margaret M. Webb, MA ~ Alive and Well, Inc.

Disclaimer: There are at least several theories of this Emotional/Social processing system. This one is called the Hierarchical System (i.e. processing moves from lower to higher). It's the one that Dr. Daniel Seigel, Dr. Allan Schore, Dr. E. James Wilder, and Dr. Karl Lehman ascribe to.

Five Levels of the Control Center*

Level One : The Thalamus	**Attachment to People**
Level Two: The Amygdala	**Attachment to Experience and Emotion**
Level Three: The Cingulate Cortex	**Attuned Connection to People**
Level Four : The R Orbital Pre Frontal Cortex	**Sense of Identity, "What it is like me to do."**
Level Five: The L Orbital Pre Frontal Cortex	**Making Sense of Experience**

* Source of the brain diagram is: www.lifemodel.org and shows only the first four levels.

BRAIN FUNCTION

When it comes to brain, the regulators for the major emotion control centers of the brain are in charge of an array of emotions such as; happiness, fear, anger, sadness, hate, shame and hopelessness. Generally, the signaling factors of controlling and regulating these emotions are very much connected to our *DNA* structure that further defines our individuality, demeanor, and our ability to relate to others in addition to the upbringing and rank in society and family. The main focus on managing the incoming data is their influence and effect on our ability to internally process and evaluate them without enduring a significant negative impact on our health and environment. Be conscious of the fact that each outcome may have positive or negative effect in our family and social fabric of our lives. Considering that each individual make processes the incoming information differently the key factor relates to our tactfulness and mastery of processing the information in a reasonable manner and minimum invasiveness. Therefore, by developing a set of processing skills to regulate our personal emotions we are building and developing a tolerance level at our brains' control center. The right side of the brain keeps an emotional regulation structure and is called the control center. Popular theory points to the first two years of life as primarily an important phase for development of the control center.

Training the Control Center

I see a correlation between the human brain and computer processor chips *(CPU)* located in center of the modern appliances and gadgets such as; television, microwave, cell phone, camera, stereo, dishwasher and car. All digital processor chips work in the same manner by loading and changing binary information which sometimes it commands to heat up a dish in microwave, other times it plays a game, trade stocks, or balances checkbook in our computer or plays music in our phone. Sometimes it malfunctions or overheats which we then either immediately identify the problem or agonize over for a while. Our control center in our right-brain is similar to a processor chip. The control center function is the same in everyone but, depending on other factors or what went wrong, control center problems can appear in different forms. Some control centers load a "bad program" and others can malfunction for lack of cooling or capacity. One person can suffer from lack of attention while another one is overly focused. One may have "out of control" feelings while another seems to have no feelings at all. One will be addicted while another may be traumatized. One may be isolated and another clingy. One may be totally oppositional and another con artist. In spite of all the differences in how these problems look on the outside, the same level of standards apply to the control center for enabling the center to perform any job which in this case the focus is on our ability to manage impulsive eating in general and over eating in particular.

My Own Experience

My favorite hobbies are quilting, knitting, and embroidery and I am equally devoted to each one of them. Additionally, for years I have been working in the technology field which requires lots of computer work with excessive typing and ultimately trickling down to excessive demand on my hands, wrists, and fingers. I paid a high price in my mid to late forties by making periodic visits to an Orthopedic Specialist for my hands and fingers. Over a period of two to three years my doctor performed multiple surgeries on my fingers in addition to one carpal tunnel correction. The routine was for me to receive two cortisone injections on each of my achy fingers for softening the callus build up in my joints before having to go through surgery. I remember waking up in the middle of the night with fingers clinched and my hands throbbing. I thought this was my new normal and sadly I thought very soon I would need to put aside my knitting and quilting hobbies since it was making my fingers and joints hurt so much. I definitely didn't want to develop deformed fingers and hands. During this period, experiencing pain in my joints became part of my daily routine and I was also experiencing pre-menopausal symptoms. My gynecologist wanted to put me on a low dose hormonal therapy to mitigate the effect of hot-flashes. Halfheartedly, I agreed to the idea but after I took the pills for five days and noticed gaining at least six or seven pounds, I angrily threw away the little tray of pills and promised myself to find another way. Coincidentally, this was the beginning of the medical discovery of hormone therapy and its potential hazards to women's health. There were rumors connecting hormone therapy to breast cancer and I intuitively felt that hormone therapy could not be a safe method altogether. So I put my thinking cap on and made a short trip to my favorite local natural herbal store and asked for advice. I found out that if I chose to take a milder gentler approach I could have an alternative method to hormone therapy. I ended up taking natural pills mainly containing Black Cohosh Root;

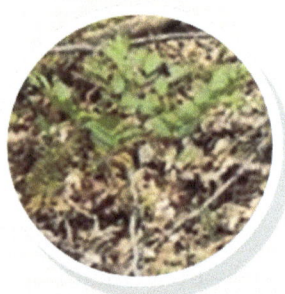 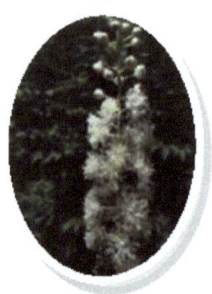

Also all B Vitamins with other natural ingredients. It did not get rid of the hot flashes altogether. However, it mitigated the effects tremendously. I also learned to manage the sudden hot flash occurrences with controlling my breathing and using meditation techniques by clearing my mind and imagining sitting in a breezy and peaceful place which proved extremely helpful.

During this period I don't exactly know what happened but I woke up one day realizing that there was definitely excess fluid in my body and I must get rid of it. It became apparent to me that the puffiness of my face every morning along with throbbing and swelling fingers was definitely related to the excess fluid. I was never a big eater so I knew it was not due to overeating.

Suddenly and without a doubt I knew who were my first and second enemies; *Salt* and without a doubt *Sugar* were my main challengers. Without further hesitation I went to work on myself by trying to correct my eating habit. At first I threw away the entire generic store bought *Morton* salts and replaced them with *Himalayan* salt. They are full of minerals and good for you when used in moderation. Concurrent to cooking with the new salt I simultaneously reduced its portion substituting the lack of salt with other spices and creative approaches. For example I added a bigger portion of sautéed onion and garlic for seasoning. I added a generous portion of turmeric and black pepper to some of my dishes.

For my spaghetti sauce recipe, in addition to other spices that recipe asks for I increased the portions of:

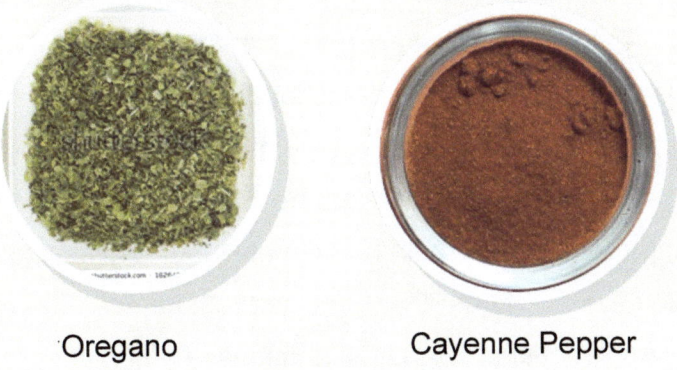

Oregano   Cayenne Pepper

I used creativity in all other dishes that I prepared and depending on each particular dish I increased the usage of:

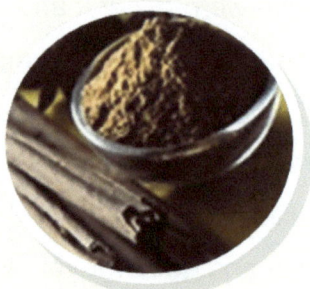

Cinnamon

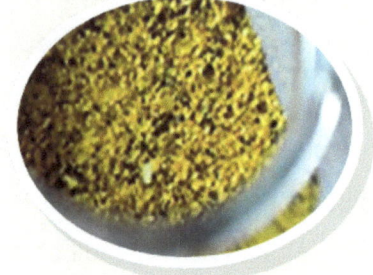

Lemmon Pepper

In addition to other yummy spices that are available everywhere. I went on to eliminate salt, sugar, and chocolate from my own food altogether. I was still eating small portions of bread and rice but not as much as before. Although I didn't seem to have any weight issue before but during this life style transformation I shed more than fifteen pounds and felt great. I also made sure to add a quality supplement from a trusted source to my daily food. As a result, I felt great, my joints stopped aching, and I could knit for hours at a time without feeling any discomfort in my knuckles. I didn't have puffy face in the morning anymore either. I felt lighter, more energetic and definitely noticed the number of my hot flashes being reduced and their impact subsided. My feeling great was such an incentive to me that I decided to take my effort to a higher level and eliminate almost all unnecessary habits as long as I could comfortably tolerate their absence. Depending on which expert opinion you tune into slamming or praising coffee drinkers I decided to continue enjoying an occasional cup of coffee but mainly drinking hot tea. To everyone's amazement not only was I not starving but was actually eating more.

Into the tenth year of what I call my sensible eating. There are no weight fluctuations. I do not experience wardrobe shrinkage and enjoy having full energy. The continuous examining and re-examining of my eating habits have become part of an effortless daily chore however, every couple of years, I have to spend a little more effort adjusting my eating to my advancing age. As time goes by I realize that it does not take too much to sustain the human body. I admit that my brain is completely adjusted to my bodily function; I can almost hear it wanting something or demanding to break away from another. This state of life may be too much to ask from everyone however, there are so many middle-of-the-road behaviors and states of mind ready to be adapted and put to work as long as we are willing to open our minds and pursue each one persistently.

Back to My Roots

My childhood was infused with daily walks to school and home; periodic walks to the local market; walks to relatives' houses who lived in close proximity to our house plus horsing around with the neighborhood kids and siblings; helping mom with gardening chores; biking and so on. This was the norm during my childhood which kept me in shape and taught me to think lean. Another typical practice on those days was to eat healthier and by that I mean beside three home prepared meals a day we were allowed to have a handful of nuts or pieces of fruits to snack on. Pastries and sweets were occasional rarities which we were allowed to have at special gatherings, birthday parties and so on. Occasionally, in long summer days if we followed our mom's instruction to the tee and finished our chores on time, we were rewarded with an ice-cream cone and that was the moment to yearn for. It is always sensible to fall back to our roots by picking and choosing the healthier and more realistic habits. After all, that series of habits were major factors forming my lifelong habits making me who I am today.

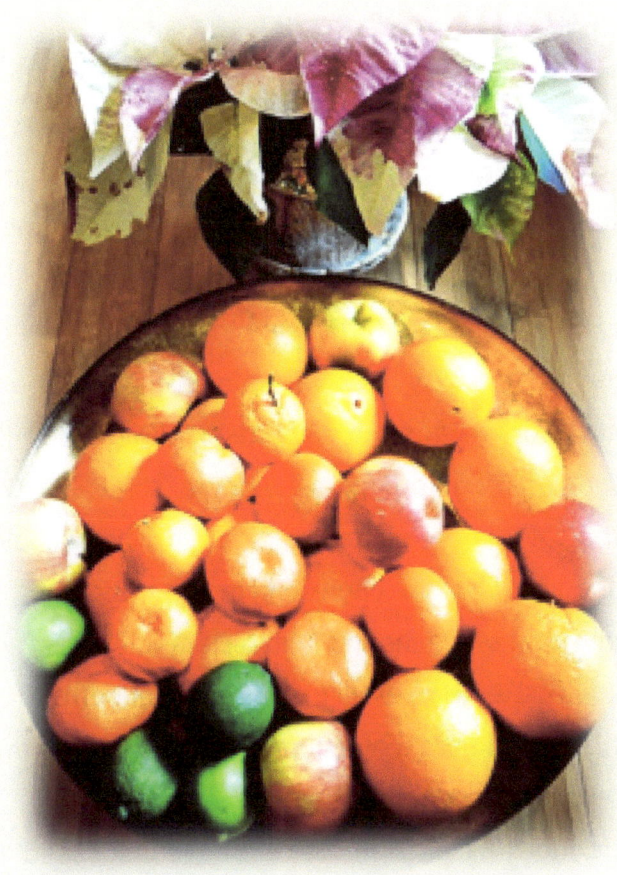

LaDan Abosein

THE FOOD WE EAT

Genetically Modified Organism *(GMO)* - What is GMO food?

You may be wondering what GMO *(genetically modified organism)* food is? It is typically referred to the food that has been tampered through genetic engineering. Starting in early 1990's some food corporations in their laboratories started experimenting with genetically modify agricultural organisms to allegedly fight the World's hunger problem. By the time the public's awareness heightened and people started to pay attention to the activists raising awareness through progressive media, scientists, & nutritionists; the creeping effect of this phenomenon was already spreading to the world of agriculture and in supermarkets everywhere with overwhelming intensity. Remember perfectly shaped tomatoes? Remember all the hype about corn which ended up with a hyped up price of corn – are you getting my point? Dr. Philip Bereano a natural health physician and *mercola.com* founder Dr. Joseph Mercola have discussed the impact of genetically modified organism (GMOs). The genetic engineering has relied on a basic fact which suggests taking out or adding one or several genes in order to create a particular outcome. However Dr. Philip Bereano a Professor Emeritus at the University of Washington and an (GM) foods and a thirty years academic and activist in Technology and Public Policy calls it the

Lego model explaining that you cannot take something out of its element and putting it into something else without wondering about further complications due to its alteration.
Source:*http://articles.mercola.com/sites/articles/archive/2011/04/02/Dr.-philip-bereano-on-gmos.aspx.*

Gilles-Éric Séralini, French scientist in his 2012 study of GMO manufactured corn experiment on rats, concluded that 70% of the female rats developed tumors and died earlier than their life expectancy. His study was published in the peer-reviewed journal *Food and Chemical Toxicology* which for the first time it unraveled the effect of *Monsanto's NK603 GM* corn treated with Roundup *(glyphosate)* herbicide for longer than 90 days on rats. *The American Academy of Environmental Medicine* has also echoed warnings. In some medical communities they discuss correlations between *Morgellons* disease which mysteriously produces sores and rashes among other issues with GMO. In the years past this controversial practice is one among many core battles between the advocates of consumers and food corporations. Despite the argument that technology can be the answer to World's hunger problem *The United Nations* has not approved the concept and the *European Union* generally bans GMO foods and imposes firm requirements on food labeling criteria.

What is Morgellons Disease?

Due to lack of serious studies and attention to the mysterious phenomenal known as *Morgellons Disease* it has been written off by many as hypochondriac mumbo jumbo. A website initiated by May Leitao in 2001 described the disease infecting her very young son. She initially called it Morgellons because the symptoms were similar to the symptoms described in a medical study during 17th century France. This is how has been described by some of its victims; strange, fiber-like material sticking out of sores or wounds that erupt on the skin. This is accompanied by painful, intense itching, that has been described as *"an ever present sensation as if something is crawling under the skin."* In 2006 local news in Oregon published a story about Dr. Drottar who suffered from the same symptoms and said; *"If I fully tell people what has gone on with me medically, they think they're in the twilight zone."* She ended up leaving her practice due to her debilitating disease.

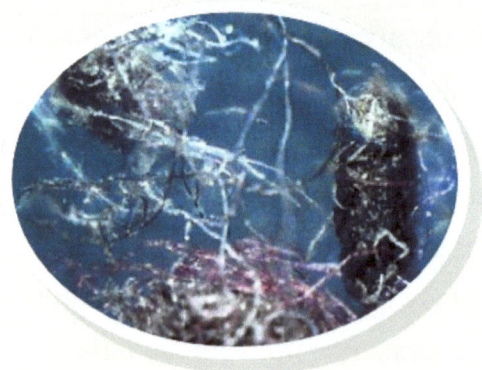

Source: *morgellonsusa.com*

The author in her March 13, 2009 article; *GMO and Morgellon's Disease* remind us of the alarming fact that due to industry, government, and media's lack of coordinated effort to push for more unbiased research on the long term effect of the GMO food

& crops on humans & animals, very little has been done which is suspicious by itself. What has happened to the inquisitive minds to try connecting the dots between the consumption of questionable food and the occurrences of some mysterious diseases? The key question to the researchers and geneticists is; is there a link between Genetically Modified Food that are regularly consumed by a person and the inorganic fibers sticking out of person's skin? The governments, who welcome GMO, have also dropped the ball by either not having proper regulations in place or not seriously enforcing them. On the global scale, the mega companies such as *Monsanto* call the shots by forcing farmers to buy their GMO developed seeds. Information has been discovered through search engines such as an article by Whitley Strieber; Skin Disease May Be Linked to GM Food concluded that *...the fibers taken from a Morgellons sufferer contain the same substance that is "used commercially to produce genetically modified plants." (October 12, 2007)*

The source for Morgellon's Disease: *http://www.rense.com*

"Genetic Engineering is a nightmare technology that has already caused MANY disease epidemics — documented but unpublicized." – Mike Stagman PhD

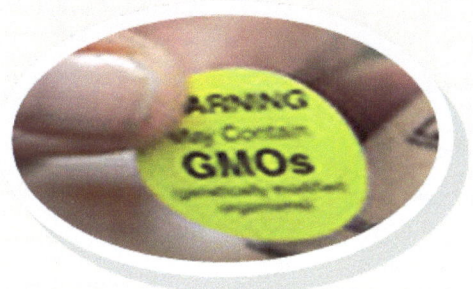

Monsanto, as part of its advertisement emphasizes that providing genetic modification with *"beneficial traits to the plant, such as the ability to tolerate drought better, resist herbicide applications or ward off pests."* They provide farmers from the GM receptive countries with seeds that; may include the following plant characteristics introduced by modifying plant's genome:

> ➤ Herbicide tolerance (Roundup Ready® crops)
> ➤ Insect tolerance (VT Triple PRO® corn, INTACTA RR2 PRO® soybeans, Bollgard II® cotton)
> ➤ drought tolerance (droughtGard® Hybrids)

Source: *www.monsanto.com/products/pages/monsanto-agricultural-seeds.aspx*
An article in *Seed Freedom.com* wrote: Genetically engineered seeds (also referred to as GMO's-Genetically Modified Organisms) mix genes in crops from unrelated organisms for example genes from soil bacteria, fish etc., which could not have mixed through biological reproduction, and conventional breeding. Two techniques via *'gene gun'* and *'plant cancer'* are used to implant a foreign gene from an unrelated organism into the plants *DNA*. In addition, antibiotic resistance marker genes or viral promoter genes are also added in this *process. The "yield" of a* GMO crop is the yield of the original plant into which the new genes were introduced.

Since most of the GM seeds are created and patented by private enterprises, farmers do not have the right to own their seeds; as result they have to buy new seeds every season. Imagine poor farmers' having to pay royalty fees in addition to the back breaking cost of seeds annually. Corporations and governments have worked out a sweetheart deal by raking in profits and passing on the excess charges to farmers and consumers. In December 13, 2006 segment of the *Democracy Now*, Amy Goodman interviewed Vandana Shiva; a prominent scholar, environmental activist, and anti-globalization author about the alarmingly high rate of suicide among the Indian farmers. Instead of paraphrasing I prefer to insert a portion of Mrs. Shiva's answer: It's something totally new. It's linked to the last decade of globalization, trade liberalization under a corporate-driven economy. The seed sector was liberalized to allow corporations like *Cargill* and *Monsanto* to sell unregulated, untested seed. They began with hybrids, which cannot be saved, and moved on to genetically engineered *Bt cotton*[1]. The cotton belt is where the suicides are taking place on a very, very large scale. It is the suicide belt of India. And the high cost of seed is linked to high cost of chemicals, because these seeds need chemicals. In addition, these costly seeds need to be bought every year, because their very design is to make seeds nonrenewable, seed that isn't renewable by its very nature,

---

[1] *Bt Cotton seeds were introduced by Bollgard Cotton, a trademark of the Monsanto group. Bt Cotton was first introduced to the U.S. in 1996 according to the University of California San Diego and was aimed at reducing the effects of the tobacco budworm and the pink bollworm. Tests began at the same time around the world on crossing the American Bt Cotton seeds with cotton produced in other countries, including India, according to the Science & Development Network. Later versions of Bt Cotton were introduced in 2003 and 2004 aimed at reducing the impact of a wider range of insects than the original version.*

but whether it's through patenting systems, intellectual property rights or technologically through hybridization, nonrenewable seed is being sold to farmers so they must buy every year. There's a case going on in the *Supreme Court of India* right now on the monopoly practices of *Monsanto*. An antitrust court ruled against *Monsanto*, because the price is so high, farmers necessarily get into a debt trap, which is why I was talking about credit, for the wrong thing, could actually be a problem and not a solution. Since there are also foreign genes in the GMO the concerning question is to know whether the crops containing GMO substance behave different from a non GMO containing crop and whether it potentially alter humans' and livestock' health. There were reports on adverse impact of *BT cotton* on human health (skin and eye allergies) from Madhya Pradesh and on livestock (cattle deaths) from Andhra Pradesh in India.

Source: *http://www.democracynow.org. & Seedfreedom.info*

It is also alarming to know that there is always a chance of the neighboring farms and crops to become affected by cross pollination mainly through natural causes such as wind patterns and traveling insects. For this and all other compelling reasons the consumers and framers must push through their governmental red tape demanding for foods to have proper labeling while the researchers, scientists, and the government through multiple studies find out the short and long term effects of the GMO food and crop.

Source: *http://seedfreedom.info/what-is-a-gmo*

The *www.criigen.org* in the Thursday 27 August 2015 article announced that: German Agriculture Minister Christian Schmidt has informed German state governments of his intention to tell the *EU* that Germany will make use of new "opt-out" rules to stop GMO crop cultivation even if varieties have been approved by the *EU*, a letter from the agriculture ministry seen by Reuters. Currently in Europe there are opposing views and discussions around the GMO crops for example; leaving Britain among those in favor of it and France and Germany among the opposition. This is different from the previous understandings that any decision approved by *EU* permits growers to farm in all *EU* states. The article refers to a deadline as to when the countries under *EU* umbrella have a chance to announce their wish to opt out of *EU* GMO farming approvals.

Source:*http://www.criigen.org/news/72/display/Germany-starts-move-to-ban-GMO-crops-Ministry-letter Michael Hogan, editing by David Evan*

GMO in drugs and vaccinations

According to Dr. Mercola most of the vaccines and flu shots contain GMO ingredients; *Chemotherapy (AKA "agent orange")* is pushed on the masses as a viable treatment for people who have been steadily consuming pesticide, fluoride, bleach, aspartame, MSG and GMO. Most developed nations do not consider GMOs to be safe. In nearly 50 countries around the world including Australia, Japan, and all of the countries in the European Union, there are significant restrictions or outright bans on the production and sale of GMO foods. Since 1990's GMO food was introduced to consumers and today seventy five percent of our food contains the product. A reasonable argument against the consumption of the GMO food is that as long as the long term effects of GMO foods is unknown and untested it is reasonable to require labeling the foods containing GMO. Then at a minimum, people who are more prone to allergies and have some kind of health problem or vulnerable people, especially babies and the elderly need to be aware of their daily food consumption. For more than decade in America, GM foods have been used mostly to feed the animals we eat. Currently, over sixty nations require labeling of genetically modified food, but not the US. American consumers are still battling at the State level to pass laws that enforce some type of labeling on food packages. However, this trend may change due to efforts taken by the State of Vermont pioneering on passing the law which requires GMO food labeling. Basically, the law requires labeling on partial or total GMO food. The law is set to go in effect July 2016 and is claimed to be the first of its kind in the US. State of Vermont; Governor Peter Shumlin indicated: *"We believe we have a right to know what's in the food we buy."* Furthermore, Dr. Mercola in his website expresses concern about the GM content vaccinations. Apparently those vaccines are already being produced and have even been recommended by the *U.S. Centers for Disease Control and Prevention's (CDC).* To reiterate my point, the key concern is lack of knowledge with the long term effect.

In 2006, researchers in the *Journal of Toxicology and Environmental Health* wrote: Genetically modified (GM) viruses and genetically engineered virus-vector[2] vaccines possess significant unpredictability and a number of inherent harmful potential hazards...Horizontal transfer of genes...is well established. New hybrid virus progenies resulting from genetic recombination between genetically engineered vaccine viruses and their naturally occurring relatives may possess totally unpredictable characteristics with regard to host preferences and disease-causing potentials....There is inadequate knowledge to define either the probability of unintended events or the consequences of genetic modifications.

Source:*http://articles.mercola.com/sites/articles/archive/2012/10/02/vicky-debold-on-gmo-vaccines.aspx*

I continue to further educating myself on GM vaccines and foods and recommend the same to everyone who is concerned about eating sensibly.

GMO and Viruses

Generally speaking, all genetically engineered crops are comprised of genetic material from viruses; packs of hereditary

---

[2] *All viruses attack their hosts and introduce their genetic material into the host cell as part of their replication cycle. This genetic material contains basic 'instructions' of how to produce more copies of these viruses, hijacking the body's normal production machinery to serve the needs of the virus. The host cell will carry out these instructions and produce additional copies of the virus, leading to more and more cells becoming infected.*

material, *DNA* or *RNA*[3] entering into the cell taking over its activities and creating a new copy of the virus. New viruses by some scientific observations; *tend to be more harmful than the natural viruses*[4]. Source: *http://www.saynotogmos.org/virus_hazard.htm*

Cauliflower Mosaic Virus (CaMV)[5]

The most common virus *DNA* used in genetic engineering is the promoter of the *Cauliflower Mosaic Virus (CaMV)* used in plant genetic engineering. it is used in almost every case, including the presently most cultivated *GE*[6] crops, the *RoundupReady (RR) Soy of Monsanto*, the *Bt-Maize of Novartis*, *GE cotton* and various varieties of *GE Canola*, a *rapeseed* variety widely cultivated today

---

[3] *A nucleic acid that contains the genetic instructions used in the development and functioning of all modern living organisms. DNA's genes are expressed, or manifested, through the proteins that its nucleotides produce with the help of RNA.*

[4] *It is notable that even the largest biotech company does not deny the possibility that new viruses may be generated. For example, Roy Fuchs, Monsanto's director of regulatory science acknowledged that "some of the virus can recombine" in an article by Stan Grossfeld in The Boston Globe (09/23/98), published on line.*

[5] *CaMV is transmitted in a non-circulatory manner by aphid species such as Myzus persicae. Once introduced within a plant host cell, virions migrate to the nuclear envelope of the plant cell.*

[6] *About 30 percent (27 million acres) of the crop in USA of 1998 is calculated to be RR Soy. Also a large crop of GE Maize has been planted (19,6 million acres). In Canada, large crops of Canola are cultivated (about 7 million acres). Every cell in the present GE crops in USA and Canada contains virus genes. One plant only contains hundreds of millions of cells. The number of plants in the GE crops in North America is altogether thousands of billions.*

especially in Canada[7]. Experiments have shown that the *CaMV* promoter may recombine with infecting genes yielding new viruses that may be more infectious than the natural viruses.

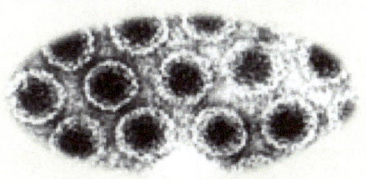

Cauliflower Mosaic Virus (CaMV)

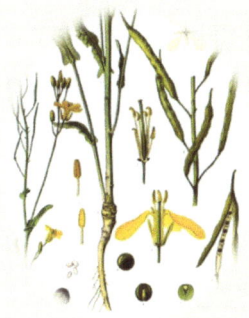

Rapeseed (Brassica napus)

Dr. Joe Cummins, Professor Emeritus of Genetics at the University of Western Ontario, Canada expresses concern and points out the fact that every plant containing hundreds of millions

---

[7] *Rapeseed (*Brassica napus*), also known as rape, oilseed rape, rapa, rappi, rapaseed (and, in the case of one particular group of cultivars, canola), is a bright-yellow flowering member of the family Brassicaceae (mustard or cabbage family).*

of cells, each containing a *CaMV* virus gene have the potential to combine with an infecting virus and ultimately generate a new virus. Furthermore, Dr. Jaan Suurkula applies the example of winning lottery to chances of a new virus being developed and indicates: Suppose there is a lottery with a million tickets. Then the chance of winning with one ticket is one on a million. But if you buy all the tickets, your chance will transform to 100% probability of winning. Every cell in the huge *GE crop* in North America is a "ticket" in the virus lottery. And there are zillions of cell "tickets" in the crop. Therefore, even if the chance for "winning" - for a new virus to turn up - would be extremely small, it may be likely to occur. Scientific laboratory experiments indicate that this probability may not be very small. To conclude with an already established fact among some scientists' that new virus resulting from recombination[8] which contains in *GE* organisms; *may become more harmful and less species specific than "natural" viruses.*

GMO in Salmon

The New York Times article called; *Genetically Engineered Salmon Approved for Consumption* (dated November 19, 2015) by Andrew Pollack: Federal regulators on Thursday approved a genetically engineered salmon as fit for consumption, making it the first genetically altered animal to be cleared for American

---

[8] *Genetic recombination is the production of offspring with combinations of traits that differ from those found in either parent.*

supermarkets and dinner tables. The approval of the salmon has been fiercely opposed by some consumer and environmental groups, which they have argued that the safety studies were inadequate and that wild salmon populations might be affected if the engineered fish were to escape into the oceans and rivers. The NewYork Times reports *AquaBounty* GMO salmon *"contains a growth hormone gene from Chinook salmon and a genetic switch from ocean pout, an eel-like creature."* Opponents say if the fish were ever to escape *AquaAdvantage's*[9] confines, they could *"out-compete wild salmon for food or mates."*

Wenonah Hauter, executive director of the group *Food and Water Watch*, indicated; "This unfortunate, historic decision disregards the vast majority of consumers, many independent scientists, numerous members of Congress and salmon growers around the world, who have voiced strong opposition." The *FDA* has not required the genetically engineered salmon to carry a GMO label, leaving that important decision to the companies whether they voluntarily label the fish as GMO product. Source*: http://www. nytimes.com/2015/11/20/business/ genetically-engineered-salmon-approved...*

---

[9] *AquAdvantage salmon is a genetically modified Atlantic salmon developed by AquaBounty Technologies. A growth hormone-regulating gene from a Pacific Chinook salmon and a promoter from an ocean pout were added to the Atlantic's 40,000 genes. These genes enable it to grow year-round instead of only during spring and summer. The purpose of the modifications is to increase the speed at which the fish grows, without affecting its ultimate size or other qualities. The fish grows to market size in 16 to 18 months rather than three years.*

In the *Common Dreams*, Nadia Prupis wrote the article; *Eco Groups Take Canadian Government to Court in GMO Salmon Fight*; Green groups on Tuesday launched a legal challenge against the Canadian government's approval of genetically modified (GM or GMO) salmon egg manufacturing, which they say was done in secret, violated environmental protection laws, and risks widespread, long-term damage. "Canadians expect government decision-making to be open and transparent, especially when it comes to something as significant as manufacturing genetically-modified salmon that may pose serious risks to wild Atlantic salmon stocks," said Kaitlyn Mitchell, an attorney with the environmental law firm *Ecojustice*. "This decision should have never been shielded from public view."*(Tuesday, November 17, 2015)*. Under then-Prime Minister Stephen Harper, the Canadian government in 2013 approved a bid by American biotechnology firm *AquaBounty* to manufacture GMO salmon eggs on Prince Edward Island *(PEI)*. From there, the eggs will be shipped to facilities in Panama and grown to adult size. A spokesperson for Canada's environmental agency said: the "risk assessment concluded that there were no concerns identified to the environment or to the indirect health of Canadians due to the contained production of these GM fish eggs." Earlier this year however, the *Canadian Department of Fisheries and Oceans* released a partially-redacted draft risk assessment (pdf) which found that AquaBounty's GMO salmon are more susceptible to certain disease-causing bacteria and are displaying inconsistent growth rates and other performance parameters. That suggests "that the growth-hormone gene construct inserted in the fish is not operating in a predictable manner, raising questions about the durability, safety and commercial viability of [GMO] salmon", the *Center for Food Safety* said in May. Source: *http://www.commondreams.org/news/2015/11/17/eco-groups-take-canadian-government-court-gmo-salmon-fight*

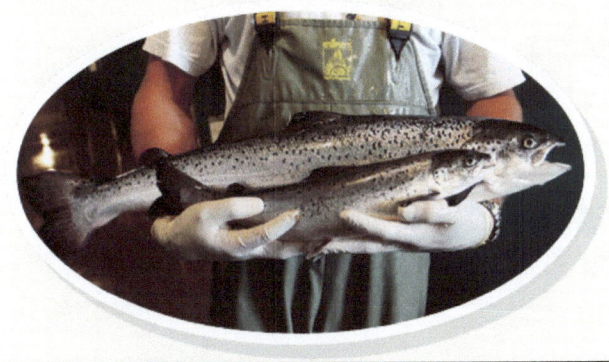

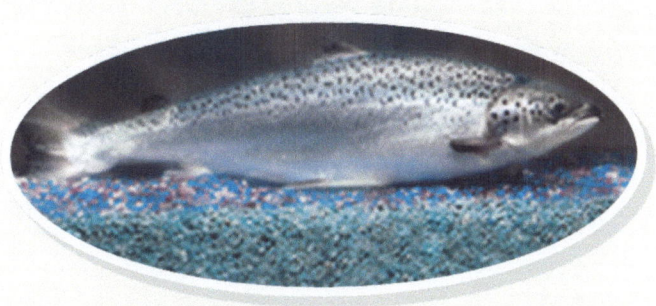

GMO in Livestock

Seattle Organic Restaurants wrote about GMO chickens' and turkeys' small cages and their intolerable living conditions which, in many cases are far from the *picture perfect* images that food corporations lead us to believe. with regard to GMO they have written; *"Chicken are GENETICALLY MODIFIED with hormones, carcinogens, GMOs, corn pills, arsenic and drugs so they become LARGER FASTER and as a result they often CRIPPLE under their own weights."* Generally, the chickens and turkeys enduring *weakened immune system* during their approximately short life of six weeks. Is there a direct or indirect correlation between the rising obesity among kids and grownups in the last decades with the GMO food? *"One out of three kids born after the year 2000 is OBESE. Consuming all these hormones, drugs, antibiotics, GMOs and carcinogens have caused chronic diseases including obesity, cancer, cardiovascular disease and diabetes".*

Source: *http://www.seattleorganicrestaurants.com/vegan-whole-foods/genetically-modified-chickens/*

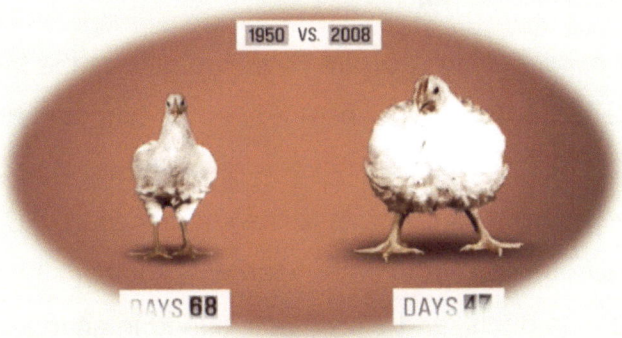

In an attempt to counter the negative press, The National Chicken Council is trying very hard to draw a rosy picture working to comfort consumers that there are no genetically modified chickens around, consequently downplaying the effect of the chicken feed which has included GMO products since 1996. Animal agriculture farmers have fed GMO corn and soybeans to their flocks and herds with the US government's blessing. The industry claim that livestock health have even improved; "*In fact, since 1996, overall chicken health has improved and U.S. production has increased by 43 percent.*" The industry is down playing the potential effect of livestock's GMO feed and brush off the labeling of chickens indicating that it does not apply to chickens since they are not genetically modified.

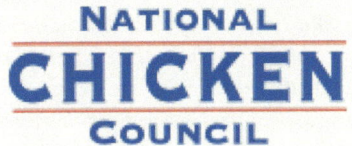

Source: *http://www.nationalchickencouncil.org/genetically-modified-organism-gmo-use-in-the-chicken-industry/*

GMO Compass, in their recent article emphasizes the fact that 60 to 90 percent of world soybeans are genetically modified and full or partial genetically modified soybeans, as the main source of animal feed arrive by ship loads to the shores of US, EU and other major ports from Brazil and other sources. Additionally, many vitamins, amino acids, and enzymes included in animal feed contain genetically modified micro-organisms that includes most medicines and vaccines used by veterinarians. According to the GMO Compass, Sausage & Ham are often genetically engineered to stabilize their oxidation process, the coloring and enhanced flavoring along with enzymes and additives that specially produced from GM soybeans or GM maize[10]. Source: *http://www.gmo-compass.org/eng/grocery*

ORGANIC AND NON-OGANIC FOOD

According to *www.helpguide.org*; the term *Organic* specifies the method by which agricultural products are grown, processed, and labeled. Organic crops must be grown in safe soil, have no modifications, and must remain separate from conventional products. Farmers are not allowed to use synthetic pesticides,

---

[10] *Maize (/ ' m eɪ z / MAYZ; Zea mays subsp. mays, from Spanish: maize after Taíno mahiz), known in some English-speaking countries as corn. A light yellow to moderate orange yellow. Maize is the only GM crop that is grown commercially in the EU. For the most part, maize is used for feeding livestock and as raw material for the starch industry. Starch, however, forms the basis of many foods and food additives. Genetically modified maize was grown for the first time in the US and Canada in 1997. Since then, GM maize production has expanded to more than 35 million hectares worldwide. Now, about 80 per cent of the maize produced in the US is genetically modified. Many countries in North and South America, Africa, and Asia grow GM maize.*

bioengineered genes[11] (GMOs), petroleum-based fertilizers, and sewage sludge-based fertilizers. Organic livestock must have access to the outdoors and be given organic feed. They may not be given antibiotics, growth hormones, or any animal-by-products. The intent of having organic food is to have food with less pesticide. Organic fruit, vegetables and live stocks that have been grown and raised locally free of GMO products, are likely fresher. The same site indicates that despite the U.S. regulatory committee's failure to require labeling on the GM food, we the consumers can still trace the source by checking the *PLU* (price lookup) code on the sticky label added to grocery store produce offering information on bananas as example:

Conventionally Grown	Organically Grown	Genetically Modified
4-digits starting with#4	5-digits starting with #9	5-digits starting with #8
E.g. Conventionally grown banana: 4011	E.g. Organically grown banana: 94011	E.g. GMO or GE banana: 84011

Organically produced crops use zero pesticides and use manure composts as fertilizers. Organic farmers use natural methods

---

[11] *The application of biological techniques (as genetic recombination) to create modified versions of organisms (as crops).*

such as crop rotation and manual weeding. For insect problems they use birds and other crop friendly insects. Contrast this with non-organic farmers, chemical fertilizers are being used to produce conventional crops, and chemical herbicides are being used to control weeds and pests. According to a nonprofit organization known as; *Environmental Working Group* that independently analyzes the results of U.S. government pesticide testing identifies certain fruit and vegetable as more susceptible to chemicals and recommends buying their organic version. Their list includes; *Apples, Sweet Bell Peppers, Cucumbers, Celery, Potatoes, Grapes, Cherry Tomatoes, Kale/Collard Greens, Summer Squash, Nectarines (imported), Peaches, Spinach, Strawberries, and Hot Peppers.* There are foods that according to the group which have higher resistance to pesticides therefore their non-organically produced kind may be as nutrient rich as their organic version; *Avocado, Sweet Corn, Pineapple, Mango, Sweet Peas, Asparagus, Kiwi, Cabbage, Eggplant, Cantaloupe, Watermelon, Grapefruit, Sweet Potato, Sweet Onions, Onions, and Papaya.* The organically raised animals and products such as dairy and eggs are raised in a chemical and GMO free environment with giving animals' free access to outdoors. The key is for the animals to live in an environment similar to their natural habitat. They may get vaccinated against diseases but they are not injected with hormones and antibiotics. In the U.S. the significant distinguishers between organic and conventional meat and dairy are: Organically raised Livestock are given all organic feed; Disease is prevented with natural methods such as clean housing, rotational grazing, and a healthy diet; Livestock and milking cows must graze on pasture for at least four months a year, while chickens must have freedom of movement, fresh air, direct sunlight and access to the outside. Conventionally raised Livestock are given growth hormones for faster growth; Antibiotics and medications are used to prevent livestock disease; Livestock may or may not have access to the outdoors.

You may look for these familiar labeling in the U.S. supermarkets:

- *100% Organic* – Foods that are completely organic or made with 100% organic ingredients may display the USDA seal.
- *Organic* – Foods that contain at least 95% organic ingredients may display the USDA seal.
- *Made with organic ingredients* – Foods that contain at least 70% organic ingredients will not display the USDA seal but may list specific organic ingredients on the front of the package.
- *Contains organic ingredients* – Foods that contain less than 70% organic ingredients will not display the USDA seal but may list specific organic ingredients on the information panel of the package.

When shopping for GMO-free food products in the U.S. and Canada, look for the Non-GMO Project Verified seal, which means that no more than 0.9% of the product is genetically engineered. *"GMO free"* or *"Non-GMO"* – without the seal, foods labeled with these terms has not necessarily undergone independent verification.

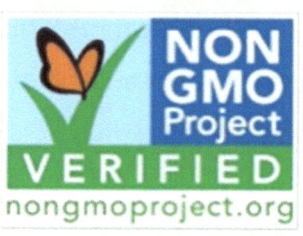　　　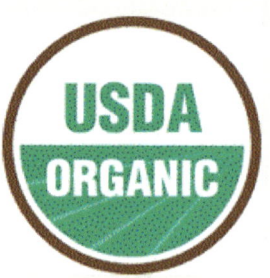

Certified Organic Food Labels in other countries:

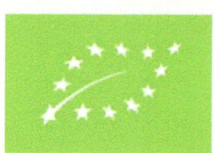　　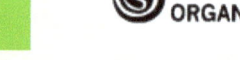　　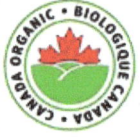

European Union　　　Australian　　　Canadian

Source: *http://www.helpguide.org/articles/healthy-eating/organic-foods.htm*

Chapter Summary

By some definitions organic foods are free of chemical fertilizers, pesticides, and preservatives produced and handled by the method defined under the *Organic Food Products Act* by *USDA* (United States Department of Agriculture). Natural food on the other hand has been referred to foods that are not chemically nor synthetically tampered with. Therefore, natural foods may or may not be organically grown and raised. Individuals, based on life priorities, style, budgets and other factors choose to eat organic or non-organic food. People like me who are not fixated with eating organic foods are nonetheless adamant about eating nutrient rich foods which, this brings me back to the subject of genetically modified organism *(aka: GMO)*, synthetically made food in laboratories that by design are wrapped in shroud of secrecy as part of a dysfunctional behavior practiced by super-sized corporations. As an example, according to *Food and Water Watch* organization, *Monsanto* has come up with a newer corn with more resistance to *Roundup*. The newer model crop has been altered to resist herbicide called *dicamba*[12] a harsh chemical that can be harmful to public and farmers' lands and crops. As chemical products such as *Roundup* become ineffective in killing weeds, corporations such as *Monsanto* develop harsher chemicals to battle the so called super weeds.

---

[12] *Dicamba (3,6-dichloro-2-methoxybenzoic acid) is a herbicide.*

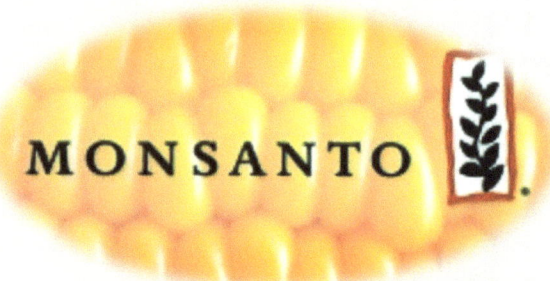

Source: *http://www.foodandwaterwatch.org/*

KEY DISCUSSION

Why there is a great public demand for sealed and certified
organic foods in America but not enough public outcry and
demand for sealed and certified natural food products?

SIMPLE EATING

Everything Salad

My bowl of salad includes almost everything under the sun and earth abundance. All the ingredients are not necessarily organic so you can use your own purchasing judgment. I cut the pieces very small allowing me to bite into a variety of ingredients with every fork full. I don't hesitate to include last minute add-ons such as pieces of fruit, pre-cooked beans or feta cheese crumbs for extra flavor and taste. For dressing, I usually use my favorite light or regular cucumber salad dressing. I periodically reduce the thickness of the dressing by adding water to the bottle which makes it easier to pour. After adding a few spoons full of the salad dressing I then top the dressing with several spoons full of one of my three favorite vinegars; balsamic, natural apple cider, or red wine vinegar. Personally, I prefer the taste and effect of alkaline vinegar to acidic lemon or lime. They both are great for the digestive system and help tremendously with the food absorption for healthy stomachs, and boost your metabolism for burning calories. The act of chewing keeps me busy for a long while; in fact sometimes I start eating my salad at the beginning of a movie and I am still chewing close to the ending.

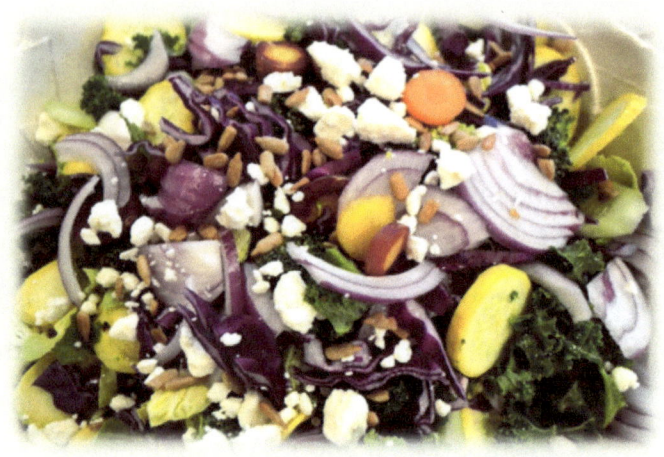

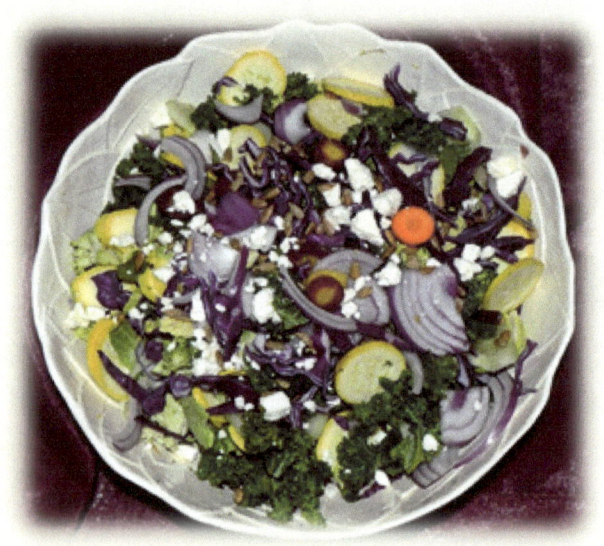

Everything Soup

Using your food processor or hands, chop off your favorite kind of vegetable add them into a large pot adding skin less chicken or vegetable broth or just water. My preference is either to cook them in water or with chicken and season with lots of turmeric and dash of salt and pepper and a few spoons of tomato paste for color. Make sure you add lots of shredded white cabbage which becomes a substitute for soup angel hair pasta and or any kind of beans of your choice. My favorite is lentil but everything works. To further enhance the flavoring at the serving time I either add a few spoons of plain low-fat yogurt or a little bit of vinegar or lemon juice to the cup. It all depends on what you crave at the moment. You may choose to eat your soup with couple of slices of toasted bread or tortilla. A gentle reminder; potatoes are starchy and somewhat fattening. I normally substitute with sweet potatoes or yams instead and add chopped kale, chard, and white cabbage for texture. You can always add pieces of chicken or turkey if you'd prefer the meaty kind. If you chose to add any kind of beans make sure to soak them overnight for diminishing their gassy effect and rinse thoroughly before cooking.

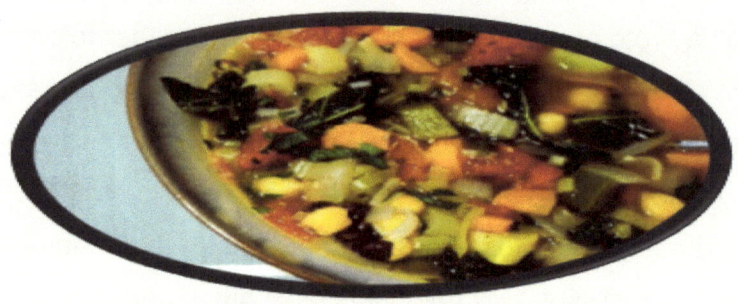

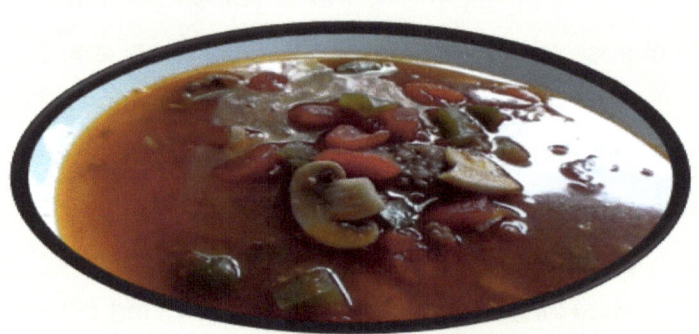

Simple Oatmeal or Cream of Wheat dish

Prepare your oatmeal or cream of wheat with tap water or nonfat milk. Chop a banana in it for sweetness and extra potassium. You can always enhance the flavor of your dish by adding Honey, raisin, and/or chopped fruit and sprinkle dash of Nutmeg or Cinnamon.

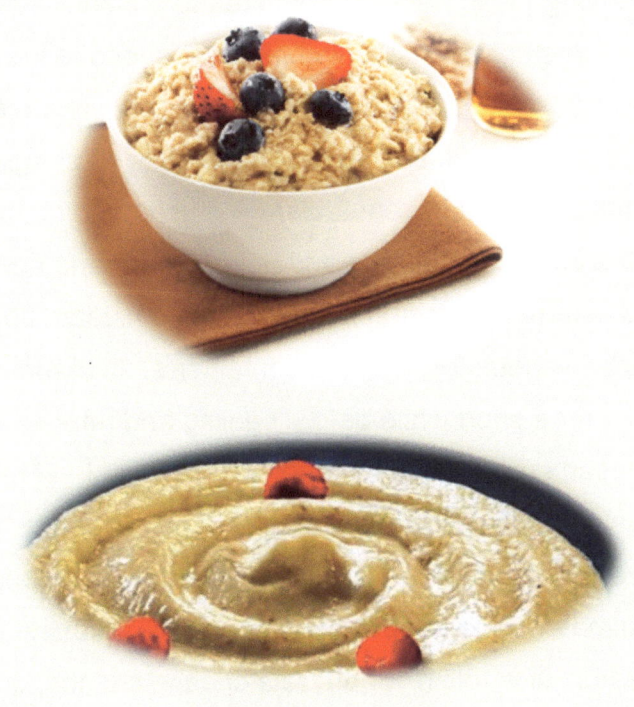

Steamed Vegetables

Cut out your favorite vegetables. Heat up a cup or two of water in a wok or a similar type of pan that holds water in the middle. Bring water to a boil in before adding your vegetables a few cups at the time. Remember not to drown your vegetable in water and add just enough to create a steam. Sprinkle a generous amount of Turmeric to your steaming vegetables. Depending on the vegetable's toughness it should not take more than 2-3 minutes to steam each batch. Use a spatula or a large spoon to transfer the steamed batch from the pan to your glass or tupperware storage container and repeat the same procedure until you complete steaming the entire cut of vegetables. Remember, you may have to repeat the process of adding and boiling water and adding turmeric to your batch several times before you steam up all of your chopped vegetables. Let the container(s) sit at room temperature for a short while before sealing and refrigerating them. You can enjoy eating them for a few days. I eat mine with salad dressing and extra vinegar on top. The vegetable has a beautiful yellow coloring (turmeric) and definitely an appealing taste. You may decide to eat it plain or add salad dressing, vinegar, lemon juice, plain yogurt, feta cheese crumbs, or similar toppings. Turmeric is very good for you and this is one of the creative ways to eat more of it.

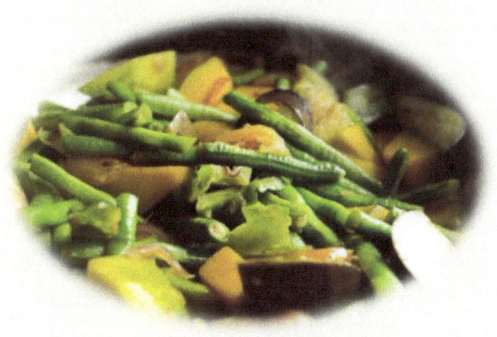

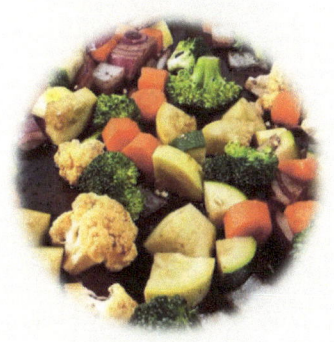

Beets

Have you experimented with beets? Try them and you may become hooked. Beets are known for their cardiovascular health benefits. Certain unique pigment antioxidants in the root as well as in its top-greens have been found to offer protection against coronary artery disease and stroke, lower cholesterol levels within the body, and have anti-aging effects.

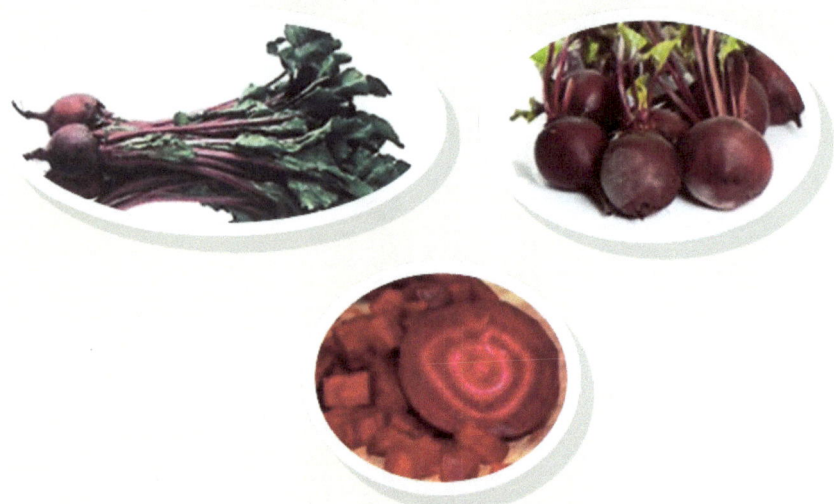

The Garden beet is known for its low calorie content with zero cholesterol and minuscule amount of fat. They are full of fiber, vitamins, minerals, and unique plant derived anti-oxidants. The root claims to have abundance source of *phytochemical*[13] compound, *glycine betaine*[14]. Betaine has been identified as a source for lowering *homocysteine*[15] levels within the blood.

---

[13] *A nonnutritive bioactive plant substance, such as a flavonoid or carotenoid, considered to have a beneficial effect on human health which also called phytonutrient.*

[14] *A sweet crystalline alkaloid, $C_5H_{11}NO_2$, occurring in sugar beets and other plants and used in the treatment of certain metabolic disorders.*

[15] *An amino acid used normally by the body in cellular metabolism and the manufacture of proteins. Elevated concentrations in the blood are thought to increase the risk for heart disease by damaging the lining of blood vessels and enhancing blood clotting.*

Homocysteine, has been identified as a highly toxic metabolite, promotes platelet clotting as well as atherosclerotic-plaque formation, which, otherwise can be harmful to blood vessels. High levels of homocysteine in the blood has been identified as resulting in the development of coronary heart disease (CHD), stroke and peripheral vascular diseases. Raw beets are known for their source of *folates*[16]. It has also claimed that extensive cooking may significantly deplete its level in food. Apparently the green leaves of the beets contain more vitamin-C and are an excellent source of *carotenoids*[17], *flavonoid*[18] *anti-oxidants*, and *vitamin A*. Beets are also credited as rich source of *B-complex* vitamins such as *niacin* (B-3), *pantothenic acid* (B-5), *pyridoxine* (B-6) and minerals such as *iron, manganese, copper,* and *magnesium.* Further benefit of the root is its moderate levels of *potassium.* I mostly eat the beets by boiling them in a pot of water. The skin will come right off when they are boiled and softened. Chop them or slice them off and mix as much as you'd like in a bowl of plain non-fat or low-fat yogurt or add a few spoons full of boiled chopped beets to your salad. For me it is the most refreshing experience and because of the yogurt I consume my

---

[16] *A salt or ester of folic acid.*

[17] *any of a group of red and yellow pigments, chemically similar to carotene, contained in animal fat and some plants.*

[18] *Any of a large group of water-soluble plant pigments, including the anthocyanins, that are beneficial to health. Also called bioflavonoid.*

daily protein too. You can also bake the beets in the oven until they are soft - a great eating experience.

Optional add-ons to a bowl of yogurt; chopped cucumber, your favorite fruit, or handful of nuts, topped off with a spoon of honey for extra sweetness. With little creativity you end up having a very healthy, colorful, and filling dinner bowl.

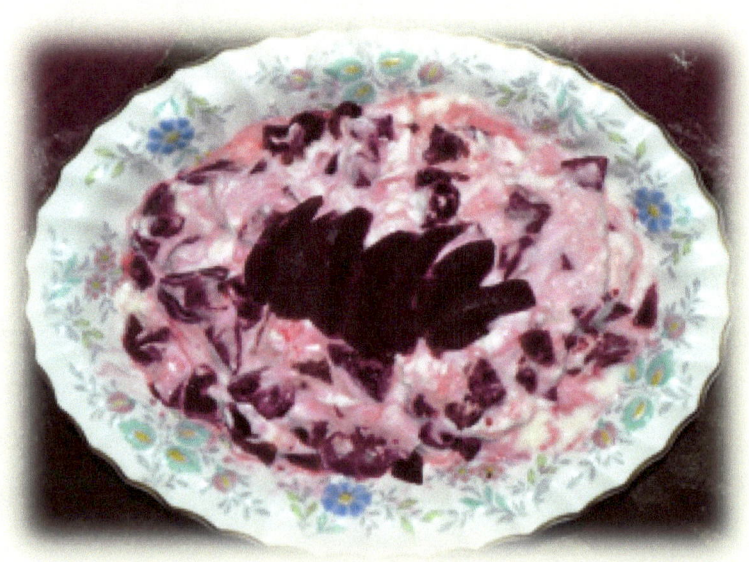

Sweet Stuff

Start substituting processed sugar with natural sugar of fruits and honey. Be aware that store bought sweet flavored yogurt is another form of low fat sugary snack without the benefit of yogurt's useful bacteria[19] and nutritional values. Enjoy eating them as snack knowing the live bacteria responsible for the goodness in plain yogurt has been tampered with since the processed sweet flavored yogurts lack nutritional value. If you'd like to eat plain yogurt and are looking for substance add your favorite fruit and nuts or honey to yogurt and make your own mixture of natural flavor. I prefer eating larger portions of low or no fat plain yogurt but some people prefer to get their healthy fat by eating smaller portion of the regular plain yogurt instead of eating larger portion of none or low fat plain yogurt.

Goodness of Nuts, Dates & Honey: The benefits of consuming these types are endless however, be aware of the high fat and calorie content in them and try exercising moderation.

---

[19] *The good bacteria in yogurt are often called probiotics.*

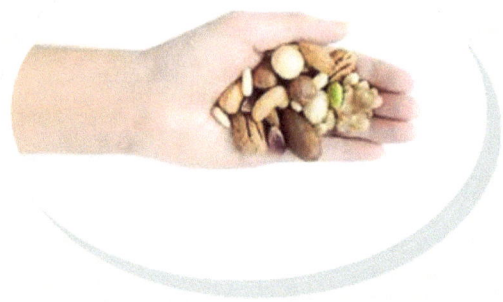

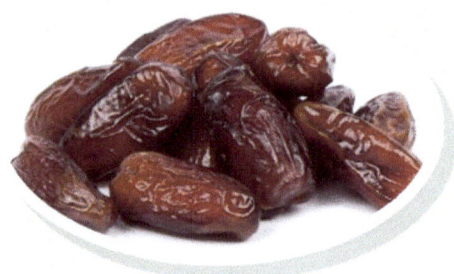

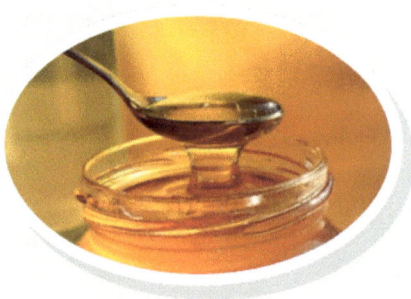

Wonders of Vinegar

For centuries vinegar has been claimed as a food and medicinal tonic. Made by the fermentation of grains such as barley, rye, wheat, and rice or juices such as grape and apple, vinegar is available in a variety of flavors and colors. Vinegar is produced by a process called distillation, in which yeasts and bacteria are used to break down carbohydrates or sugars. Medical studies have already proved the health benefits in vinegar with essential nutrients that are important for healthy digestion, food metabolism, and energy production. All vinegars are beneficial for heart, blood vessel, nerve, and healthy muscle.

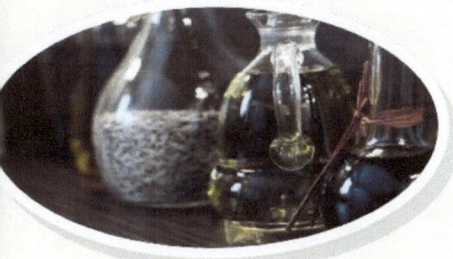

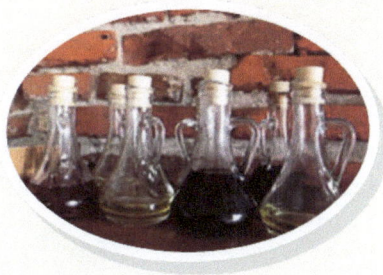

Benefits of Turmeric

According to popular belief Turmeric contains anti-inflammatory properties and turmeric extract is effective in reducing pain caused by osteoarthritis. Turmeric may also help reduce eye inflammation and gum disease. A daily intake may reduce kidney inflammation and lower blood pressure. Products that contain curcumin such as turmeric may reduce itching and irritation resulting from skin wounds and rashes. Turmeric is a ginger-like plant whose roots are gathered, dried, and made into a spice for flavor and health benefits. The scientific name of turmeric is *Curcuma longa*. The turmeric spice that you buy in grocery stores is the boiled, dried, and powdered root of the turmeric plant.

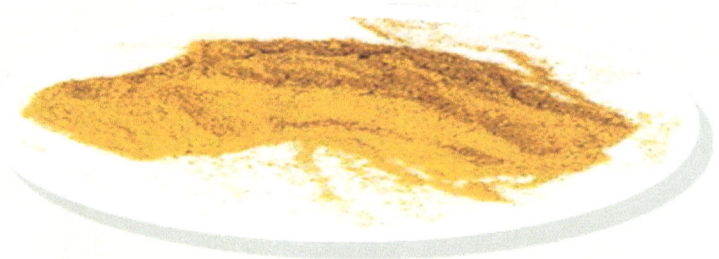

BONUS RECIPE

Home-made pickles

In the past twenty plus years I have been making my own pickles. It has become such a rewarding summer activity for me that I never can picture myself reaching for a jar of pickles at the grocery store. Over the years I have perfected my own method without having to follow any particular recipe. I like them to sound crunchy and taste spicy sour with touch of sweetness. I prefer to use more vinegar and less water, a variety pickling spices and less salt and finally I use freshly washed and dried pickles instead of blanching or pre-boiling the pickles[20]. By using my method of cleaning and drying the vegetables and bathing the jars I have avoided an oxidation problem and my pickle jars have been stored for years without losing their freshness and crunch when opened. Lately, my challenge has been keeping them on the shelves to last until the next summer batch is made – a real tribute to the chef.

General instruction

I am not the exact measuring type; rather leave the measuring to individuals based on their pallets. Every summer around the mid-August or early September I look for the best pickles and pickling ingredients at the farmers market or stores dedicated to zealous pickling enthusiasts.

---

[20] *Blanching method is performed by two minutes of boiling the vegetable and one minute of dipping into the ice bath.*

For approximately fifteen to twenty pounds of pickling cucumber

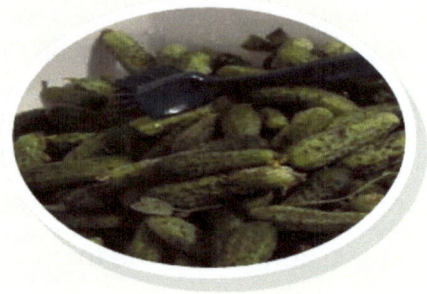

I use three one gallon jugs of apple cider vinegar

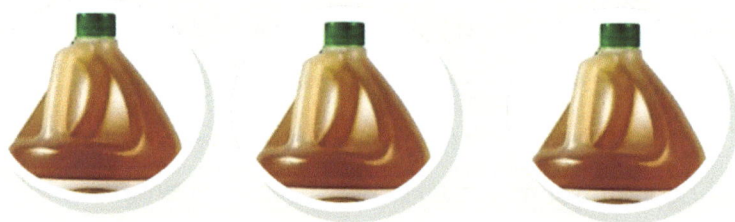

Two bunches of fresh dills for their flowery ends

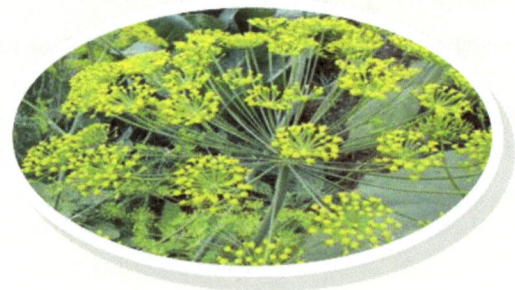

At least six pounds of mild, medium, & hot jalapeno peppers (adding one of each in every jar makes the pickles spicy and for a milder effect you can eliminate the smaller hot pepper)

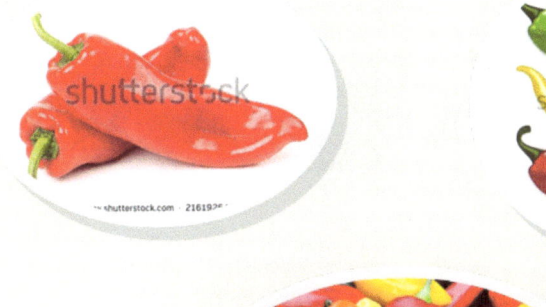 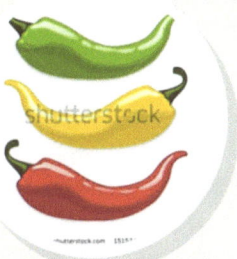

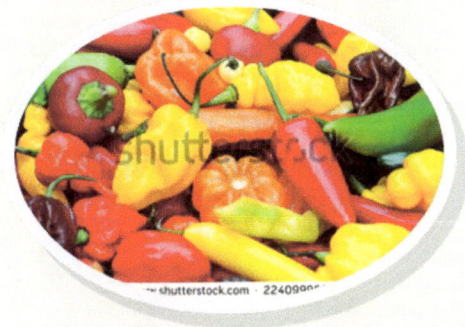

Twenty medium size whole garlic

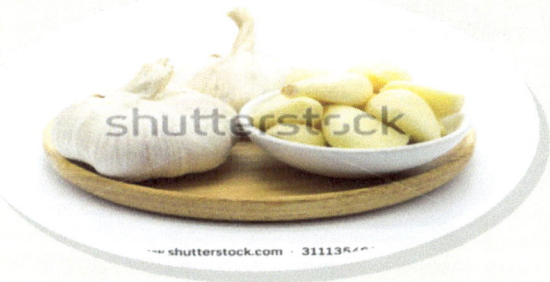

Two bunches of fresh mint; two bunches of fresh tarragon (if in season)

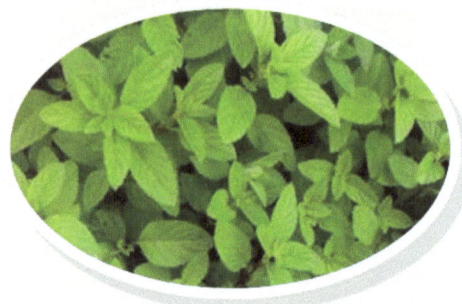 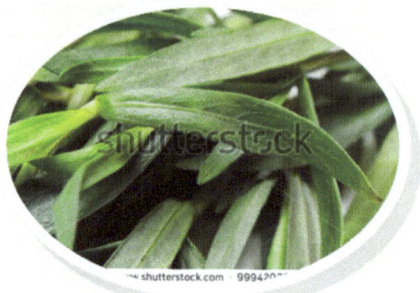

One or two pounds of mixed pickling spices, dried dills (if available), salt, & sugar

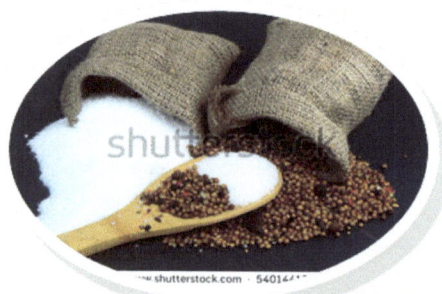 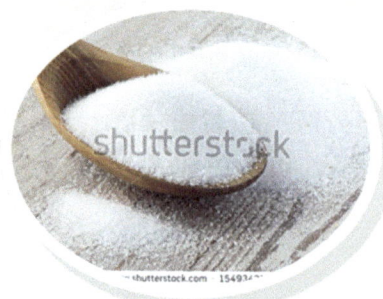

I make sure I have 20-25 quart size glass jars and the lids, cleaned and ready nearby

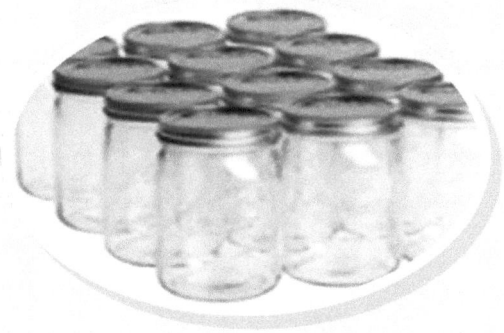

I use two large deep pots; one for boiling the jars and one for mixing the ingredients

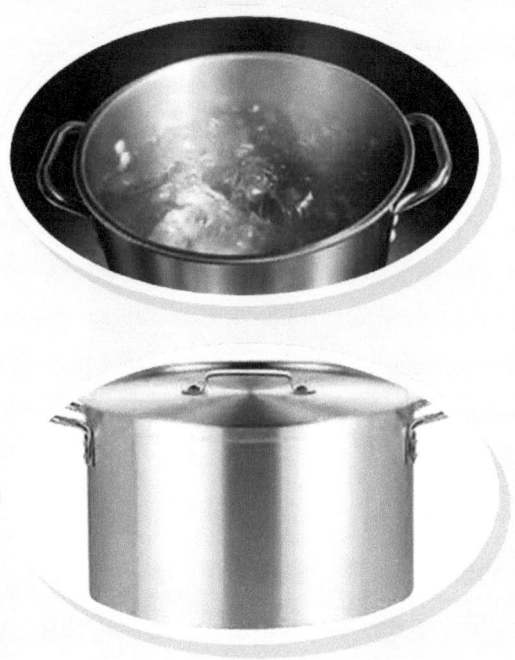

A key to having pickles that can stand the test of time without losing their freshness is to eliminate their exposure to oxygen. To make this happen you must wash and dry everything thoroughly. By that I mean washing every pickle and vegetable thoroughly by hand and drying just as thoroughly. The jars must be completely dried after the boiling process. Make sure you have plenty of clean and dry towels and working surfaces. Peel the garlic into cloves. Arrange all the ingredients in an orderly manner on a table or a counter top and get ready to boil the juice and the jars. Empty the vinegar into a large deep pot, add the spice mixture to the pot with salt, turmeric, and sugar (to your taste). You may use kosher, Himalayan or pickling salt and just enough sugar to subside the sour taste of vinegar. This recipe is almost similar to the sweet and sour pickles but with less sugar. Start boiling the ingredients and while stirring you can adjust the flavor to your taste. Simultaneously, start boiling the jars and lids in a large pot of water and remember to repeat this sterilization process until all the jars are sterilized. Use tongs or rubber gloves to handle the jars when you are removing them from the boiling pot of water and clean towels to dry each jar's inside, outside and the lids. Make sure you have plenty of clean towels at your disposal. Once the jars are dried and while they are hot or at least warm start packing them with pickles. My ritual is to throw a few cloves of peeled garlic to the bottom of the jar, add one or two mint or tarragon stems, one or two dill flowers, and one spoon full of dried dill, then arrange the pickles and add one of each jalapeno peppers upright and very tightly packed. Finally, if your jar has any extra room fills it with a couple of extra garlic cloves and mint stems in between the pickles. Pack the jars as tightly as you can. By now you should have a pot with hot ingredients. Remove the pot from stove and put it next to your jars. Using a medium size wooden or sturdy plastic ladle, fill each jar with the hot mixture and make sure that each jar has fair amount of pickling spice mixture. Each jar should be filled to the rim with juice. When the jars are full, clean the excess juice from around outside of each jar with a clean towel. Using a flat plastic or wooden spoon press any remaining air bubbles out of each jar then close each jar with the two piece lid. Now you are ready for the water bath process.

In the same pot of water that you used to sterilize your jars, place the filled jars with their lids closed in an upright position. Depending on the size of the pot you may manage bathing four to six jars at a time. The water in the pot needs to be at least up to the middle of jars. Cover the pot and boil them for fifteen to twenty minutes. Remove the jars and repeat the same process until you have run all of your jars through the water bath process. Place the jars on a cool or room temperature surface until they are cooled down. Make sure to press each lid with your fingers and tighten the lid again. You may hear a popping sound which means the excess air is bursting out. After a few hours you can transfer you're cooled down jars to your pantry or shelves that are away from heat or excess sunlight.

Important Note

ONLY use wooden or plastic spoons during the pickling process.
Stay away from anything that oxidizes such as metal utensils.
You DO NOT want to expose the jars and ingredients to any
moisture that can enter into the jars. Pickling process is intense
and for making twenty-five or thirty jars of pickles be prepared to
spend seven to ten hours in the kitchen.

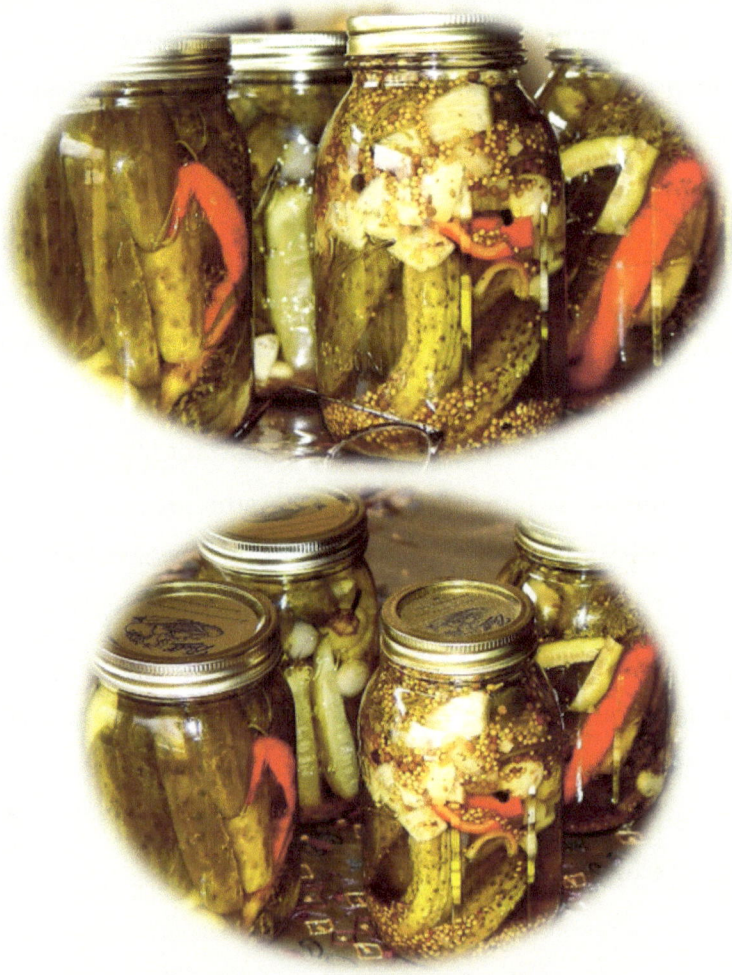

ABOUT THE AUTHOR

LaDan Abosein moved to United States in the 70's where she earned her Bachelor degree in Psychology from Purdue University and Master's degree in Organizational Development and Management from Webster University. LaDan raised her family and built her career working in High Tech industries. She has always been passionate about making things right. She always looks forward to visiting her daughter and granddaughter; Isabella *(Bella)*.

www.ingramcontent.com/pod-product-compliance
Lightning Source LLC
Chambersburg PA
CBHW050809290526

45792CB00001B/47